Shadow Walkers

Author: Peter T.Raven

This book I write for those of us that had one or multiple strokes, or other brain damages since I think we all pretty much feel the same way or at least many of us do.

My name is Peter and I had a severe stroke back in 2012 July 21st.

I remember it like it happened yesterday and I know that the aftermath will

follow me to end of my
time here.

When The stroke hit I was
in financial drop down and
had lost my apartment and
practically lived in my car
for several months.

And the basic needs I used
the gas stations or truck
stops to be able to shower
and wash my clothes and so
on.

Not the ideal living but was enough to stay alive.

I am at present 50 years old and the stroke hit me at age 46.

I am the father of four boys and when the stroke happened I had been visiting my two next oldest we had spent the day with inline skating and also bike riding and when we returned to their home I felt very strangely tired.

Sure we had been spending
a lot of energy during the
day but I was rather well
trained and fit in body so
this just felt strange to me I
should not be this tired after
the activity's.

But actually I did so I
excused myself and drove
my car to a remote location
to try to get me some rest.

When the car was parked I
placed myself in the rear

seat of my car a Volvo
station wagon.

I fell asleep instantly and
slept very deep for many
hours.

I woke up by my cell phone
someone had text me and I
half sleep tried to fix my
eyes to read the text it was
my next oldest son 16 at the
time asking if I was awake?

I thought I wrote him back
yes I am now and pressed
send.

He responded with plenty
question marks.

I thought I wrote him the
same answer again and
once again he returned
question marks to me.

I tried to sit up better in the
back seat and put my leg in
pressing state but nothing
happened.

Then I noticed that my right
arm had fallen to the car
floor and I lifted it back up
on the seat thinking my
awkward position had made
it fall asleep.

Now my son was calling
me and I answered the
phone and he asked what I
was doing?

I answered that I had just
woken up very blurry so he
said what?

My right arm had once
again fallen to the car floor
and I tried to lift it up but
absolutely nothing
happened.

Now I got scared and
worried I have worked in
medic care and this seemed
very familiar to me.

I tried to force my right leg
to the car floor to sit myself
up but nothing happened.

I tried to speak clearly to
my son.

I said you need to call for
an ambulance I think I am
having a stroke.

My young son got scared
and handed the phone to his
foster father and I repeated
that I needed an ambulance
quickly and he asked me
where I was and I gave him
my location.

He answered we are closer
we come and pick you up
and the call was ended.

My only thought was that I
had to get outside the car
right now to the cool air.

I used only my left side of
my body and kicked and
dragged myself out from
my car and tried to stand
upright leaning to my car
gripping the roof list and
hold on as hard as I could.

My body just wanted to lay down and just end to function I knew my life depended on that I stayed standing.

The cool air made my mind a bit clearer but I now noticed my fascial paralysis in full effect the right side was gone I felt nothing.

Finally, I saw car lights approaching they were here at last.

My son came rushing
towards me with the tears
running and he tried to
support me but I was
simply too heavy for a 16-
year-old boy.

His foster father drove his
car closer and then he
gripped around me and
placed me in the back seat
of his car and then we
speeded towards the
hospital.

During this period of time I went in and out of consciousness and my sons foster father yelled at me to stay awake and to keep talking but I just couldn't.

I don't remember the car trip completely but I remember seeing pictures from the past when my sons were small and when I married my ex-wife and such my body prepared to close down.

When we arrived at the
emergency intake my sons
foster father had called
ahead and told them we
were coming so the crew
was on standby.

They quickly put me on a
stretcher and rolled me
away for treatment.

Well this is my own
personal story of the event
that day and it is all very
true and still kind of hard to
think about still.

I have been told far after the
stroke moment that I was
actually arriving just in time
to be saved 15 minutes later
I would have died all
according to the treating
doctor.

So now four years after I
still asking myself
questions like what if my
son didn't text me that night
what then?

If I had not dragged myself out from the car to the cold air what then?

As many of you can probably conclude it would have killed me for sure.

So I must say I am very grateful to still be alive and be able to support all of my four sons and actually I was given this talent to write books after the stroke so I can share my stories with you.

Well this was my own story of the event but I would like to talk more about what me and many others like me are actually thinking and feeling today.

I can of course only talk about my own thoughts and feelings no one else's.

For me everything after the stroke moment changed my personality completely and not for the better sadly.

The first period of time
after the stroke I felt
completely helpless just
lying in a bed not able to
move around much and not
able to speak due to the
fascial paralysis.

But inside my head there
was heavy activity I felt
what is the point? What do I
have to live for? I have no
goals anymore just let me
die.

These were my actual
thoughts and I can say that
some still remain in my
head today.

I was ready to give up I saw
no reason to stay alive at
all.

The doctor examined me
and told me that I would
never walk again due to the
gravity of the damages done
inside my brain.

This was the spark I had
been waiting for hearing
him say I would never walk
again set my soul on fire
and woke my inside
warrior.

I wrote to the doctor on a
piece of paper that I will
walk again and I will talk
again and also drive my car
again.

The doctor smiled and
responded calmly that is not
very lightly and he said

don't set up such high
hopes.

He left my room and his
words was stuck in my head
how dared he?

That moment I remember
so well since that was the
moment I decided to fight
for survival I will prove that
fool wrong.

His words still remain in
my brain I will never forget
his words to me.

These words have been my motivation and the spark to the inside warrior to never ever give up and aim for the stars.

And I can reveal to you all that now four years later I can talk again not only Swedish but English very well to.

I can walk again without any support and best of all I regained my freedom and drive my own car again.

But I won't lie the path here
has been very hard and
many times I wanted to just
give up and die.

The doctor's words kept me
going the past few years
and I have proved him
wrong in everything he told
me and that feeling is so
satisfying really.

Sure I still have issues to
work on I can't do balance
taking activities at least not
yet.

But I struggle each and
every day to get stronger
and to move forward in my
fight to regain my own
body.

Many in the hospital staff
and also my training helpers
think my progress this far is
beyond any expectations
and sure I have moved
forward pretty good but I
am not satisfied until I
control my own body again
that is my goal.

It is my body it should obey my commands without and fuzz.

Well after the stroke my personality have changed I wrote earlier let me explain a little about that to.

My emotions are not the same as before I don't feel anything special at all an example is during my own rehabilitation my mother passed away in terminal cancer and sure me and my

siblings was at her side on
the hospital and yes I was
some kind of sad but I
didn't cry I only felt
emptiness nothing normal
grieving emotions and I
can't tell you why since I
don't have an answer.

When my stepfather died
also from terminal cancer I
cried and was sad for
almost two years after his
passing but that was 13
years ago before the stroke.

A very recent event was when my biological father died December the second last year 2015 I felt nothing at all and I loved my father once upon the time.

So my emotions are very messed up after this close call and I have been told by my own family and my siblings that I am a completely different person these days I don't care for love I don't socialize I

don't show any emotions
what so ever.

And yes maybe that is the
truth I feel pretty much the
same but I always have the
feeling I left a big chunk on
the other side not all of me
returned from the death
threshold.

It is a very strange feeling
and is extremely hard to
describe to normal people
but I am doing my very best
here.

These days I don't feel in
the same way as before I
don't behave as I used to
people that have known me
for more than twenty years
don't know who I am
anymore.

Well I am sorry this I can't
do anything about what
returned is who I am today
and I may appear as very
cold and without any
emotions what so ever and I
have extremely hard to

show any emotions
happiness sadness pain love
I just don't remember how
to I am sorry but this is who
I am.

Let me try to explain who I
was before the stroke if that
is alright with you.

When I was younger in my
teens I was very popular
along the girl's community

And I had many girls
chasing me around and I

loved to have girls around me.

I was often out with my friends partying and simply enjoyed life and at the age of 28 I met my ex-wife and she was only 18 when we met and soon enough we had our first son and the next followed a year later and the third one year thereafter so we struggled with three toddlers and the life was great.

Son number four arrived
five years later and we were
a large and happy family.

But we can jump in time
until my ex-wife started to
cheating on me and soon
got very heavy drinker of
alcohol that finally lead to a
drug abuse in form of
amphetamine and that was
the end to that marriage of
obvious reasons I was home
managing the kids and she

was out partying around all over.

Oh well that is past time we divorced and walked in different directions that is now eight years ago and my ex-wife now is free from drugs and alcohol at least I think so.

We don't keep that close contact anymore and actually I don't keep anyone close to me anymore.

And my economy went
from bad to worse and I lost
my apartment and ended up
living in my car as I told
you before.

And after my stroke
incident my ex-wife visited
me once in the hospital
during my rehabilitation
and my two oldest boys
visited me maybe two times
each during my four-year
rehabilitation so family
support not very lightly.

And you need to keep in mind during these four years of rehabilitation I lost my mother and my biological father and these events didn't help much in my own struggle to remain alive.

I can honestly say that every day I look for some sort of reason to get out of bed and perform this day to satisfaction to myself and my boys but you should know that it is getting harder and harder to motivate myself to keep going.

Many days I catch myself thinking why? What is the point? And so on still and I try to find some kind of motivation to keep going and at present it actually is my book writing that keeps me going there is so many stories I want to tell you but sometimes I just lack the inspiration to write things down.

So if this should happen at least you all know the reason why I went silent and don't publish any new work.

Good back to the book title the Shadow Walkers what I mean with this title is that I and many with me walk around on the streets but actually many of us are not present at all.

Sure we look as any other person on the street we maybe act like most people but there is a big difference between us since I know myself that I feel like I am completely out of place I don't feel like I belong here.

After my own stroke I feel like I actually died on that summer day of July 21st and everything after that point is

like living on borrowed
time it's not the life I had.

This person that I face in
the bathroom mirror each
day just isn't me I feel like
a stranger in my own body
like I said it is very hard to
explain the way I feel and
how I look on myself today.

It feels like I am an empty
Wessel just drifting on the
ocean of time without any
destination and without any
goal.

Today I just drift along and try to find any meaning to roll out of bed in the morning I don't really know how I can explain it any clearer than that and trust me I am really trying to make you understand how I and many with me are actually feeling after being this close to death.

This was not my first encounter with death actually it was my tenth encounter in my life but that is a different story.

What I can say is this after every close encounter with death you always leave something behind and in my own case I actually wonder how much still remain of the original person Peter?

Well actually I don't really know how to answer that since I have absolutely no clue what so ever.

But this existence I am
living is so very different to
who I was and I don't feel
emotions in the way they
are supposed to be shown
many of my friends ask me
what do you feel about me?

Sadly, I can only respond
that I actually don't.

That answer is far from
what they want to hear I
know but should I pretend
to feel something that I
actually don't?

Nah I always try to be frank
towards people and sure
many times my responses
can be hurtful and for that I
apologize but I can only
reply what I actually feel
right?

I think I remember what
love feels like and also
anger so actually they are
both very basic feelings but
I think I remember love
since I have my four sons
and I have my ex-wife that I

spent almost half my life
together with.

But if I remember how it
actually feels to fall in love
again?

Well I am sorry to say I
actually don't know but
maybe someday that special
someone appear in front of
you and then I guess I
would know if I could fall
in love again or not.

I care for many people
around me but love is a
powerful word so I am very
careful how I use it these
days.

But the anger then?

Yes, the anger follows me
like the pain in the butt and
every day I try to think in
some kind of happy
thoughts or happy events
from the past that put a
smile on my face.

My long term memory is a
bit splitter and sometimes I
mix happenings together
and some events I even
wonder when did these
actually happen?

Where did they happen?

Who was there?

Everything is a mess at
times

And I do my very best to
keep them sorted but I don't
always succeed.

So this anger can attack at any time sudden noises a person says the wrong words to you maybe a fellow driver approach you to fast or don't show where they are going with the turning signals and so on it can be so many things that trigger this angry behavior but for the most times I am very calm since I have some blood pressure issues as is rather common in my age.

And I also use nitro spray at
ocation to keep the pump
working I only wished there
could be a shop online
where you actually could by
a new freshly restored brain
and do an upgrade on
myself.

That would actually be
awesome to get everything
working in perfect balance
again but as far as I know
there is no such on line
shop for human upgrades.

Yes, my friends I think this
will conclude this book
since I don't actually know
what else to talk about for
now at least.

Maybe some of you other
people with similar issues
recognize yourself in my
book maybe not but I hope I
have delivered the message
loud and clear to all of you
readers and remember all is
not what it appears to be.

Regards Peter.

www.ingramcontent.com/pod-product-compliance
Lightning Source LLC
Chambersburg PA
CBHW070229290526
45789CB00004B/1544